CMO

CETYL MYRISTOLEATE

A NATURAL TREATMENT FOR ARTHRITIS AND OTHER JOINT-RELATED DISEASES

RITA ELKINS, M.H.

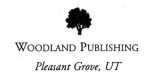

WOODLAND PUBLISHING
Pleasant Grove, UT

© 1997

AirEau
Books

European & UK Distributor:
**AirEau Fittings Limited,
Heathcote House, 1 Heathcote Road,
Bordon, Hants GU35 0BN.
Tel: 00 44 (0) 1420 473383 Fax: 00 44 (0) 1420 476140**

CONTENTS

INTRODUCTION

Physicians have been prescribing the same arthritis treatments for decades. They have been using steroid drugs like cortisone and NSAIDs as their primary therapeutic agents for joint inflammation, and the side effects from these treatments are considerable. While new pharmaceutical drugs are emerging that help regenerate cartilage, they come with a number of deleterious side effects and, like cartilage surgeries, are still considered radical therapies.

Today, the focus of arthritis treatment has turned from simple symptom relief to actual joint intervention. In other words, natural compounds which help to heal and protect the joints rather than simply mask the pain caused by their deterioration are considered superior therapies. Cetyl myristoleate (CMO) is one of these compounds and it has some impressive credentials. It is considered nontoxic and is currently the subject of widespread interest because it appears able to mitigate joint destruction through its involvement with the immune system.

Called the "arthritis immunizer," CMO has recently come to the forefront of natural osteoarthritis remedies as an effective substance capable of not only treating inflamed joints, but protecting them from further destruction as well. It is considered a natural and safe compound that has shown efficacy in treating people who suffer from osteoarthritis, rheumatoid arthritis, and the type of joint inflammation associated with psoriasis. CMO is classified as a nutrient and is considered nontoxic. Clinical studies conducted on CMO support its use as a pain reliever in cases of joint inflammation. The rapidity with which it takes effect, coupled with the permanency of its therapeutic effects after a relatively short course of treatment, makes it well worth investigating.

The need for an effective, accessible and safe supplement designed to treat osteoarthritis is significant. Therapies designed to restore the viscosity of joint fluid, inhibit the inflammatory response, and to help regenerate cartilage tissue are the types of treatments which will eventually overcome debilitating forms of arthritic disease.

A Technical Definition of CMO

CMO is a medium-chained fatty acid which liquifies at approximately room temperature and resembles a yellowy oil at 98.6 degrees (body temperature). At cooler temperatures, the lipid compound becomes a waxy substance. It is a naturally occurring substance which is absorbed in the intestines after being ingested orally. It can be extracted from living tissue or produced synthetically. CMO occurs in certain mice species, male beavers and sperm whale oil. Currently, it is being produced synthetically without using any animal extracts.

Chemical Analysis

CMO is a fatty acid ester known as cis-9-cetyl myristoleate and can be technically written as: $CH_3 (CH_2) 15OCO (CH_2) 7CHCH (CH_2) 3CH_3$. This fatty-acid compound consists of both single and double bonded chemical types, including both medium and short chain molecules. CMO is a lipid which is characterized by the presence of fatty acids or their derivatives. Lipids are essential constituents of practically all plant and animal cells. They are composed of five main elements: carbon, hydrogen, oxygen, nitrogen and phosphorus. CMO can technically be considered a waxy lipid.

A BRIEF HISTORY

CMO became the subject of scientific inquiry when researchers at the National Institutes of Health discovered that certain species of laboratory mice were protected against developing adjuvant (induced) arthritis. Harry Diehl, who worked in the Laboratory of Chemistry of the National Health Institute of Arthritis and Metabolic and Digestive Diseases, is credited with the actual discovery of CMO. In the 1960s he initiated a number of experiments designed to identify cetyl myristoleate. These studies and others found that a particular family of mice possessed a biological compound capable of protecting them against the development of arthritis. This compound, known as cetyl myristoleate, was subsequently isolated through gas chromatography and mass spectrophotometry.

Scientists theorized that this specific substance acted as a joint protector against induced arthritis. Consequently, a double blind study ensued where ten male rats were injected with CMO and nine control rats received nothing. All of the test rats were then given an injection of *Mycobacterium butyricum,* also known as Freund's adjuvant. The rats that received the CMO injection remained completely free of joint swelling or inflammation. By contrast, the other nine rats experienced major symptoms of arthritic disease (Diehl 1, 296).

Further study confirmed that animals who were given prior injections of CMO and then exposed to arthritis-producing agents did not develop the disease or any of its symptoms. Diehl, who himself suffered from osteoarthritis, used the compound himself and reported permanent success. A paper on CMO was subsequently published in the *Journal of Pharmaceutical Sciences* discussing its apparent ability to completely protect against arthritic disease (Diehl, 296).

CMO is now available for purchase in the United States and is classified as a nutritive supplement. A patent was issued under the name of cetyl myristoleate in 1996 to Harry W. Diehl of Rockville, Maryland. Earlier patent documents disclose that originally CMO's primary purpose was to protect against and treat forms of rheumatoid arthritis. Subsequent patents were issued supporting the use of CMO for osteoarthritis as well. Interestingly, an earlier patent referred to the compound as a way to "immunize" against rheumatoid arthritis.

Cetyl myristoleate is currently marketed under several brand names. Over the last several years, CMO has been used in numerous cases of both rheumatoid and osteoarthritis with some impressive outcomes. Full remissions of pain and inflammation have reportedly occurred after taking CMO for as little as two weeks.

CMO: Arthritis Immunity?

In an important research study, ten normal Swiss albino mice received an injection of Freund's adjuvant, an arthritis-producing substance. Within a period of ten to twenty days, no swelling was observed in the legs or paws of this group of mice. This implied that this particular species of mice possess some type of protective compound that works against arthritis. Consequently, scientists did tests on these mice and were able to isolate the CMO compound. To test its efficacy, developed a double-blind study using rats instead of the protected mice. In this study ten rats were given an injection of CMO and then 48 hours later received the arthritis-inducing agent. A control group of nine rats received the Freund's adjuvant alone. Both groups were observed for fifty-eight days. Every one of the rats that received only the Freund's adjuvant developed severe swelling of their front and hind legs, neglected to gain weight and exhibited general malaise. Those rats which had been given the CMO, on the other hand, showed no evidence of swelling and grew over five time faster than the other rats. It was concluded that CMO afforded complete protection against adjuvant-induced arthritis in rats. (Diehl, 296-99). Cetyl myristoleate has been referred to as the "immunity factor" because it afforded laboratory test rats such protection.

While CMO was originally extracted from mice tissue, recent technological advancements have made it possible to successfully synthesize the compound in the laboratory. This process requires a series of complex chemical reactions, making it costly to produce. Today, the synthetic production of CMO has been expedited, making it possible to purchase the compound without using animal sources.

It is important to note that experiments have found that the purer the concentration of CMO, the more dramatic the results. Patent reports detailing the ability of CMO to protect mice and rats from developing the symptoms of rheumatoid arthritis attest to the scope and potential of the compound in human beings.

OSTEOARTHRITIS: A DEBILITATING DISEASE

Arthritis may be the oldest and most treated disease in the history of mankind. For generations, tonics and potions with the promise of curing this debilitating disease have been created and readily sold. Most people who suffer from arthritis are willing to try just about anything to remedy its miserable symptoms.

Arthritis is characterized by an inflammation of the joints

9

with accompanying pain, swelling and stiffness. Osteoarthritis typically strikes older people, and is the most common form of arthritis. It affects over 80 percent of people over the age of fifty. Statistics indicate that over forty million Americans suffer from some degree of osteoarthritis. It is the leading cause of physical disability in the United States.

Typically it is our weight-bearing joints which are most affected by osteoarthritis, as well as the joints of our hands. The course of the disease involves progressive cartilage destruction and hardening, followed by the formation of bone spurs in joint cavities. Without the presence of healthy cartilage, our joints lose their "shock absorbers" and become vulnerable to wear and tear. When joint protection is compromised, joint and bone damage results along with subsequent partial or complete immobilization and sometimes deformity. Something as seemingly innocuous as cartilage is what enables us to move freely and without pain.

CAUSES OF OSTEOARTHRITIS

While rainy, damp weather does not cause arthritis, it definitely seems to aggravate the condition. Osteoarthritis may be caused by a number of age-related factors including an altered biochemistry which causes a decline in certain biocompounds and hormones. This condition typically attacks the knees, hips, and fingers and occurs when cartilage cushions which line the joints become stiffer and rougher. Consequently, bone can actually overgrow the joint area which causes swelling and decreased movement. In its final stages, arthritic pain may actually subside, but by that point the joint will have become totally immobile. Heredity may also play a factor in determining who is susceptible to developing osteoarthritis. The following list summarizes factors that influence the development of osteoarthritis:

- age-related changes in collagen synthesis and repair
- fractures or other trauma to bones or joints
- genetic predisposition
- altered biochemistry due to other diseases or foreign substances
- hormonal dysfunction
- excessive wear and tear
- inflammatory joint disorders

SYMPTOMS

In its initial stages, the symptoms of osteoarthritis can be very mild and hardly noticeable. Joint stiffness in the morning is often the first symptom of the disease. Arthritis may be limited to only one joint or may affect many. Initially, one may notice that after a certain activity a joint may feel sore. With time, pain, stiffness and limitation of use occur. Depending on the joints affected, the symptoms of arthritis can vary somewhat. The following symptoms are typically experienced during the course of osteoarthritis:

- early morning stiffness
- swelling
- recurring tenderness in one or more joints
- changes in the ability to move a joint
- redness or a feeling of warmth in joint
- creaking and cracking of joints
- edema and pain that worsen the more the joint is used
- deformity (in severe cases)

STANDARD MEDICAL TREATMENT FOR OSTEOARTHRITIS

The class of medications called NSAIDs (nonsteroidal anti-inflammatory drugs) are some of the most widely prescribed drugs in the United States—a fact which strongly suggests that pain has become a way of life for most Americans. Unfortunately, because of their accessibility and the free manner in which these drugs are prescribed, they are taken liberally for everything from a slight headache to severe arthritic pain.

Aspirin, along with several other drugs, is an NSAID. Traditionally, it was used to treat the pain and inflammation of arthritis. While it may be effective during the initial stages of the disease, when the condition worsens very large therapeutic doses are required. Such doses often create toxic side effects, including a ringing in the ears, gastrointestinal irritation, and blood thinning.

Today, other NSAIDs are commonly prescribed by doctors for arthritis. They include: ibuprofen (Advil, Nuprin, Motrin etc.), indomethacin (Indocin, Indometh, Naprosyn), fenoprofen (Nalfon), and meclofenamate (Meclomen, Meclofen). While these types of NSAIDs may be better tolerated than aspirin, they are not necessarily more effective. In addition, they are quite costly and pose significant health risks when used over long periods of time and in certain dosages.

Using corticosteroids has also been a traditional treatment but poses even greater health risks. Steroid drugs should only be used as a last resort in cases where a physician has determined that they are absolutely necessary. Ironically, long term use of steroid drugs can weaken bone structures and actually cause arthritic-like conditions in some people.

SIDE EFFECTS OF NSAIDS

NSAIDs come with a host of undesirable side effects. Prolonged use of this particular class of drugs may actually hasten the progression of arthritic disease. Certain studies have shown that NSAIDs inhibit the process of cartilage repair in that they impede the synthesis of collagen matrix (Newman, 11). Ironically, the disease mechanisms which cause osteoarthritis are actually boosted by the use of NSAID drugs. The fact that some studies strongly suggest that the use of these drugs may actually accelerate cartilage destruction is extremely significant but rarely addressed by medical practitioners. Most people who suffer from osteoarthritis are not aware of this particular undesirable action.

Other side effects associated with NSAIDs include stomach upset, stomach ulcers, liver damage, kidney dysfunction, dizziness, tinnitus, lowered blood sugar, and abnormal heart rhythms. In addition, taking ibuprofin can increase the action of sulfa drugs, phenytoin, phenobarbital and anticoagulants. Anyone with kidney trouble or who is pregnant or nursing should not take NSAIDs without their doctor's approval. Mixing alcohol with certain NSAIDs can also be dangerous. Millions of people take NSAIDs daily and thousands suffer related side effects. By contrast, a CMO protocol offers significant therapeutic benefits for arthritis sufferers without the deleterious side effects of NSAIDs and steroid drugs.

FATTY ACIDS AND ARTHRITIS

It is fascinating to learn that one of the few natural sources of CMO is sperm whale oil, a substance that has been traditionally touted for its medicinal properties. CMO is a lipid-based compound comprised of Omega-3 fatty acids. Omega-3 acids, found in some cold water fish, constitute some of the best natural anti-inflammatories available and are highly recommended for arthritis. Evening primrose oil, black currant oil, borage and flaxseed oil contain gamma-linoleic acid (GLA) which is also good for joint inflammations. Numerous clinical studies support the efficacy of GLA in the treatment of arthritis. Tenderness, stiffness and joint inflammation have decreased in a significant number of patients receiving essential fatty acid treatment. Specific fatty acids have the ability to mitigate decreased joint inflammation by boosting the production of prostaglandin E1, a powerful anti-inflammatory agent.

CMO is a medium-chained fatty acid with single-double bonded types. Its chemical signature explains why it turns into a waxy state at room temperature and an oil at body temperature. While it does not technically fall into the category of the EFAs, the fact that it belongs to the fatty acid class of compounds implies that it may have similar anti-inflammatory properties. In addition, CMO seems able to manipulate immune response, which explains why it has been referred to as a "joint protector." The fact that it is found in sperm whale oil suggests that it may have a function similar to the cold water fish oils which have significant therapeutic effects for joint inflammations.

HOW CMO WORKS

When CMO is taken in oral form, it is absorbed through the intestinal tract and migrates via the blood stream to joint receptor sites where it becomes attached. While the exact physiological mechanisms involved in CMO therapy are not fully understood, it appears that this compound actually alters the immune system response that triggers joint inflammation and causes pain and swelling. The presence of CMO within affected joints seems to block the inflammatory response, resulting in a cessation of pain and a decrease in swelling.

Arthritis triggers inflammation, an immune reaction which initiates the release of certain compounds and biological processes which cause redness, pain, and the accumulation of fluid or edema. While this response can be good for infections, allergic reactions, autoimmune diseases and arthritis, the process works to injure and destroy tissue rather than to salvage it.

CMO has the unique ability to mitigate and inhibit inflammation in body joints. It provides a shield of sorts against this immune response with amazing efficacy and longevity, even after a relatively short period of administration. Simply stated, CMO has the ability to inhibit the symptoms of arthritic disease and is also considered an immunizing agent against the development of rheumatoid arthritis.

FORMS OF CMO

CMO can be compressed into tablet form or can be encapsulated into a hard shell capsule or soft gelatin capsule. It is also available in oil form and can also be found in ointments and salves for topical application. CMO is also available in various arthritis formulas or as a liquid elixir. It can be administered orally, topically or parenterally. Look for high potency, pure products with a minimum of filler or vehicle substances.

STORAGE RECOMMENDATIONS

Keeping CMO supplements at room temperature is acceptable if the environment is dry. It can be refrigerated but it will turn into a solid substance at colder temperatures.

15

SAFETY

Tests on CMO-containing products have found no side effects or toxicity. CMO should be given to children only when under the supervision of a qualified health care provider. Its effects on pregnant or nursing mothers has not been studied. Individuals suffering from liver disease or asthma should not take CMO without the approval of their health care professional. In fact, anyone who is contemplating CMO treatment should consult their physician. As is the case with any fatty acid supplement, care should be taken to use the product in recommended doses only.

HOW TO TAKE CMO

Generally, a CMO protocol involves a three to six week course of treatment. A minimum of thirty days is recommended for maximum efficacy. Some individuals notice an improvement after ten to fourteen days; however, other may require up to six weeks or more to see desired results. Therapy typically involves taking a recommended number of capsules or liquid several times a day with a break of several days, with a resumption of treatment until the entire amount of CMO has been consumed. The proper dosage of CMO should be based on body weight and the severity of the arthritic condition. Typical amounts range from 0.05 to 0.075 grams of CMO per 140 to 200 grams of body weight.

If breakthrough pain occurs, treatment can be reinitiated. CMO appears to protect the joints for an indefinite period of time even after treatment has stopped. Some reports indicate that breakthrough pain occurs in a small percentage of CMO users after they have initiated treatment. Advocates of CMO believe that this is a positive sign that the supplement is taking effect. This assumption is based on the idea that when CMO targets affected or diseased joints, it causes a reaction with accumulated waste products of inflammation. It is believed that with continued treatment, this pain will subside. One of the most impressive attributes of CMO therapy is that prolonged treatment with the compound does not appear to be necessary in order to maintain therapeutic effects. (NOTE: If you have trouble digesting and assimilating fats, taking lipase may help to ensure the proper absorption of CMO, a fat-based compound. Taking fat-absorbing supplements like chitosan may interfere with the proper assimilation of CMO.)

TESTIMONIALS REGARDING CMO THERAPY

A number of testimonials are circulating regarding the benefits of CMO therapy. While considered nonscientific, anecdotal surveys contribute to the overall documentation of CMO as a credible treatment for joint diseases. These testimonials include a number of success stories, some of which have been condensed into the list form below. Also included are examples from the patent documentation.

ORAL CMO THERAPY

- knee pain and swelling gone after years of trouble
- neck motion greatly improved
- heel spurs disappear
- shoulder arthritis greatly improved; pain free and good mobility
- immobilized fingers regain motion and flexibility
- back surgery avoided in cases of spinal stenosis

- hip pain alleviated
- liver inflammation decreased at same time CMO therapy was initiated
- manual labor with arthritic hands possible after therapy
- leg stiffness alleviated and cholesterol levels dropped
- lung capacity improved simultaneously with symptoms of neck arthritis
- two week therapy with CMO alleviated pain from rheumatoid arthritis
- pain in hands, feet, shoulder and neck gone after a three day therapy
- wheelchair-bound arthritic patient restored to mobility after two week treatment
- pain caused by accident trauma to hip was alleviated within twenty-four hours
- morning foot pain gone with two day treatment

TOPICAL APPLICATIONS OF CMO

- hand eczema that still existed after eighteen years of steroid cream application cleared up
- alleviation of back pain with solutions of CMO applied on the skin

PATENT REPORTS

1. A 250 pound, 75-year-old male diagnosed as suffering from osteoarthritis received four 1 cc capsules of CMO orally two times, with about a two month interval between the dosages. The result was at least a 75 percent alleviation of pain in the afflicted joints. Only minimal pain persisted following medication in the lower back and hips, and the knees, elbows and other joints were almost completely pain free.

2. A 72-year-old male diagnosed as having osteoarthritis took three capsules of 1 cc of cetyl myristoleate, followed five months later by four more of the same capsules. His osteoarthritis was sufficiently alleviated that he was able to discontinue other arthritis medication and resume playing the guitar.

3. A 65-year-old female suffering from osteoarthritis received four capsules containing 1 cc each of cetyl myristoleate orally. She experienced complete recovery from the osteoarthritis within a short time of taking the medication (U.S. Patent #5569676).

In addition, several other reports on CMO treatment disclose success with painful football injuries, knee surgery recoveries, hand gripping problems, finger swelling, hip injuries, decreased hand dexterity, consistent aches and pains. There is only anecdotal evidence that CMO may also be beneficial for the type of joint pain associated with gout and other nonarthritic diseases; however, the possibility exists that CMO may help inhibit the type of joint inflammation associated with autoimmune diseases like lupus.

CMO: RAPID AND EFFECTIVE

Believers in CMO therapy are passionate about its amazing properties and the rapidity with which it takes effect. Some have gone as far as to claim that it is 98 percent effective against both osteo- and rheumatoid arthritis. While more study is certainly warranted, anyone who suffers from arthritis should inform themselves about CMO therapy. Consult your physician.

PRIMARY APPLICATIONS
OF CMO

- osteoarthritis
- psoriatic arthritis
- lupus
- back pain
- joint injuries
- Reiter's Syndrome
- autoimmune diseases
- ankylosing spondylitis
- rheumatoid arthritis (several reports claim that CMO is also effective for rheumatoid arthritis as both a preventative and therapeutic agent)

BIOENHANCING AGENTS

Several other nutritional supplements exist which serve to augment CMO therapy nicely. These are all substances which have documented therapeutic properties for the treatment of joint inflammation. Anyone who suffers from arthritis or related diseases should incorporate a nutritional strategy based on the use of certain dietary supplements and foods.

Ideally, CMO therapy should be a part of a nutritional regimen designed to boost its overall effectiveness. A completely natural approach to osteoarthritis is preferable and addresses several factors which contribute to joint damage. Anytime the body is faced with a healing crisis, nutrition must be considered as a major player in promoting tissue repair and preventing further destruction. In addition, certain herbals and other substances can augment nutrition and enhance overall health. Specific vitamins, herbs and other constituents specifically complement CMO and speed healing.

GLUCOSAMINE SULFATE

Glucosamine sulfate is a naturally occurring amino-monosaccharide found in highly concentrated amounts in the joints of mammals. When taken as a dietary supplement, glucosamine appears to be able to significantly restore normal biochemistry in supporting the rebuilding and healing of osteoarthritic cartilage. It is an ideal supplement to proper nutrition because it supports cartilage function and repair over extended periods of time with no toxic side effects (Setnikar, 243).

The body recognizes glucosamine as a natural substance and does not react to its presence in a negative way. It does not artificially suppress or stimulate normal cellular function, but rather augments physiological processes which have deteriorated with age, causing the gradual destruction of cartilage stores. Ideally, glucosamine should be taken with chondroitin sulfate.

CHONDROITIN SULFATE

Chondroitin is a chemical compound comprised of a long chain of sugars. It is a natural compound which is found in some dietary sources such as certain animal tissues. Dietary chondroitin will usually become assimilated in various body cells (i.e. cartilage tissue). The long chemical chains of chondroitin react with the spine of proteoglycan molecules located in cartilage areas of joints. This reaction forms spaces within cartilage allowing for much better water retention and protection.

The chemical structure of chondroitin helps to create a watery shock-absorbing space within cartilage tissue. In other words, chondroitin helps to enhance the fluid protection of joint systems, resulting in better lubrication and nutrient transport. When fluid accumulates in this manner, cartilage that is usually destroyed by arthritic disease stays more flexible and exhibits greater strength. Chondroitin has the unique ability to draw in and retain the fluid that cushions our joints and makes them mobile. In addition, chondroitin is able to inhibit the action of specific enzymes which breakdown cartilage tissue and contribute to its destruction (Rovetta, 53-57).

Apparently, other enzymes also exist which can prevent the proper transport of vital nutrients to cartilage tissue. Chondroitin interferes with them as well, giving cartilage the opportunity to stay intact and well nourished. Moreover, chondroitin can stimulate the synthesis of proteoglycans, collagen and other cartilage molecules which contribute to the production of new cartilage cells.

VITAMIN C WITH BIOFLAVONOIDS

Because vitamin C plays such an integral role in collagen synthesis and connective tissue regeneration, it is crucial to any regimen designed to treat arthritic conditions. Vitamins C and E work in tandem to enhance the structure of vital cartilage constituents and are thought to prevent or minimize the deterioration of cartilage.

VITAMIN E

Some studies have found that vitamin E can benefit people suffering from osteoarthritis (Machtey, 328). It has proven antioxidant action and actually works to inhibit the breakdown of enzymes found in cartilage and enhances cartilage regeneration.

OMEGA-3 OILS (FISH OILS)

Fish oils contain Omega-3 fatty acids which provide substantial amounts of vitamin D, necessary for proper bone growth and function. Fish oils compete with certain fatty acids that trigger arthritis inflammation in cases that are not age-related. These oils are high in vitamin A which may act as a natural anti-inflammatory.

FLAXSEED OIL

Flaxseed oil is full of essential fatty acids and has been linked to a number of beneficial effects including decreased cholesterol, heart health, and treatment for inflamed joints.

SHARK CARTILAGE

Cartilage extracts can be obtained from both bovine and shark sources. Shark cartilage contains certain compounds known as mucopolysaccharides or glycosaminoglycans. One of the constituents of these molecules is chondroitin sulfate, which is actually comprised of chemical units of glucosamine sulfate combined with sugar.

Studies conducted at the University of Miami School of Medicine found that arthritic pain could be substantially decreased by using shark cartilage extract. Dr. Jose Orcasita, M.D., stressed the fact that patients who took shark cartilage for arthritis experienced no side effects or toxicity of any kind. Those he tested using shark cartilage experienced significant improvements (Gagliardi, 52).

Apparently shark cartilage targets arthritis in two ways: first, it acts as a natural anti-inflammatory to ease joint pain; and second, it helps to prevent the growth of an abnormal network of blood vessels that can develop in inflamed areas. The presence of these vessels significantly contributes to the pain and stiffness associated with arthritis. Bovine cartilage and colostrum have also been used to alleviate arthritic joint inflammation.

BORON

Supplements of boron have been utilized in Germany as a treatment for osteoarthritis for over three decades. A recent double-blind study evaluated its effectiveness and found that of patients who took six milligrams of boron, 71 percent experienced improvement as opposed to a 10 percent improvement rate seen in the placebo group (Traverse, 127).

METHIONINE

This amino acid has proven its ability to rival the therapeutic effects of ibuprofen in treating the pain typically present in cases of osteoarthritis. The sulphur content of this amino acid is thought to support cartilage constituents, including protoglycans and glycosaminoglycans.

CALCIUM WITH MAGNESIUM CITRATE

This very absorbable form of calcium and magnesium helps to fortify bones and works to prevent the bone loss that can sometimes result from advanced cases of osteoarthritis.

DEVIL'S CLAW

Devil's claw (*Harpagophytom procumbens*) is a botanical which is indigenous to regions of Africa. It has quite a lengthy record of use for arthritis and has recently come under scientific scrutiny.

Clinical studies involving animal models have found that devil's claw possesses an anti-inflammatory action that rivals phenylbutazone, a powerful synthetic drug. Devil's claw is more effective for the treatment of osteoarthritis than for rheumatoid arthritis. (*Note:* Some studies exist which dispute the anti-inflammatory action of devil's claw. It would only stand to reason, however, that if native Africans used this botanical as a traditional treatment for arthritis, the usage must have its basis in effectual therapeutic mechanisms.)

CAT'S CLAW (UNA DE GATO)

For generations, Peruvians have trusted the anti-inflammatory attributes of cat's claw. Historically, it has been used for arthritic joint conditions. Clinical studies conducted on the plant metabolites of cat's claw have discovered that it does inhibit the inflammatory response. The plant sterols found in the herb exhibit the ability to reduce artificially induced swelling in the paws of rats (Aquino, 453). Cat's claw also contains a source of proanthocyanidin, a phytochemical which acts as a potent antioxidant (De Matta, 527). Because proanthocyanidins (sometimes referred to as pycnogenol) scavenge free radicals so effectively, they have shown some remarkable curative effects. Regarding arthritis, proanthocyanidins have proven their ability to significantly reduce joint inflammation.

YUCCA

Yucca extracts have been successfully used as part of an arthritis protocol at the Desert Arthritis Clinic. Some health practitioners consider yucca as a natural precursor to synthetic cortisone. This makes it useful in controlling swelling and inflammation.

BOSWELLIA SERRATA

Modern medicine and pharmacology are just beginning to realize the value of this ancient natural substance. *Boswellia,* a gum resin which is harvested from large trees native to India, has significant antiarthritic properties. Also referred to as "salai guggul," this resin contains an acid which has shown its ability to control arthritis in a number of animal studies. Among its actions are the ability to inhibit inflammation through interfering with inflammatory mediators, the improvement of circulation to affected joint tissues, and the prevention of a drop in glycosaminoglycan levels (Singh, 407). Studies point to this resin as a potentially viable treatment for both osteo- and rheumatoid arthritis. No side effects or contraindications have been reported with *Boswellia serrata.*

GREEN BARLEY JUICE

Green drinks made from green barley contain a whole array of nutrients, including superoxide dismutase, an enzyme that helps to destroy the free radicals that damage the synovial fluid needed to provide adequate joint lubrication.

WHITE WILLOW (*SALIX ALBA*)

This natural substance is extracted from white willow bark and is rich in salicylates, natural anti-inflammatory agents that reduce swelling and redness and are useful for joint and muscle pain.

CAPSAICIN OINTMENTS

Clinical tests have confirmed that topical capsaicin ointments made from cayenne pepper can substantially alleviate the miserable pain that characterizes osteoarthritis and rheumatoid arthritis. Ester Lipstein-Kresch, M.D., has studied the effectiveness of capsaicin creams for arthritis and recommends applying it three or four times a day on the affected areas for at least two weeks. An initial burning sensation at the site is not unusual and will subside with continued use.

PROANTHOCYANIDINS (PYCNOGENOL)

For joint injuries and arthritic conditions, proanthocyanidins (pycnogenol), which are extracted from grape seed or pine bark, act as powerful anti-inflammatory compounds without any of the negative side effects associated with over-the-counter or prescription drugs. Proanthocyanidins bind with collagen fibers and help to alleviate arthritic pain and swelling. They are considered much more powerful in their antioxidant action than vitamins C and E.

RECOMMENDED FOODS

Foods rich in bioflavonoids are recommended and include blueberries, blackberries and cherries. In addition eat plenty of high fiber, whole grains. Phytochemicals such as sulfur are also good and can be found in onions, garlic, cabbage and Brussels spouts. Fresh raw fruits and vegetables contain live enzymes and are all recommended—with the exception of those belonging to the night-shade family: potatoes, peppers, tomatoes and eggplant. All legumes including lentils, split peas and beans are good, as well as fish and most seafood. (NOTE: Some studies have found a link between low sulphur content and arthritis (Travers, 127). Supplementing the body with doses of sulphur has been successful in some cases of arthritis for pain and swelling. What these studies suggest is that eating a sulphur-rich diet and using sulphur supplements may be a great benefit for people with arthritis. Interestingly, glucosamine sulfate naturally contains sulphur compounds.)

FOODS TO AVOID

Foods to avoid are fatty red meats, sugary rich foods, dairy products, egg yolks, soda pop, saturated fats, and, in the opinion of some experts, vegetables considered part of the nightshade family. These include tomatoes and eggplant. Also avoid dried fruits, salted nuts and eliminate tobacco and nicotine.

CONCLUSION

Fortunately, compounds like CMO are gaining the type of attention and focus needed to bring them to the forefront of therapeutic options available for people who suffer from arthritis and other joint-related diseases. When a person is the victim of the type of pain associated with arthritis, knowledge of what's available is crucial. More and more people are turning to natural alternatives for the treatment of diseases like arthritis. Unfortunately, many who suffer with chronic pain have come to rely exclusively on pharmaceutical drugs which may control pain but do little to promote healing.

CMO is a natural compound that holds some very exciting possibilities and treats the pain and inflammation typical of arthritis in a unique and beneficial way. Its ability to block the arthritic inflammatory response is undisputed. While physicians may be slow to advocate its usage until more studies emerge, CMO's promise cannot be put on hold. As is the case with any new medicinal compound, care must be taken to know the facts, to obtain reliable products, to use them correctly, and then to draw a personal assessment of whether or not the compound is effective. People who suffer from osteoarthritis and its related diseases are entitled to the facts and should be given the opportunity to draw their own conclusions.

REFERENCES

Aquino, Rita, et al., "Plant metabolites, new compounds and anti-inflammatory activity of *Uncaria tomentosa.*" *Journal of Natural Products*, 54 (2), Mar-Apr. 1991, 453-59.

De Matta, S.M., et al., "Alkaloids and procyanidins of an *Uncaria* species from eastern Peru." *Farmaco-Sci*, 31 (7), July, 1976, 527-35.

Deihl, H.W., "Cetyl myristoleate isolated from Swiss albino mice: an apparent protective agent against adjuvant arthritis," *Journal of Pharmaceutical Sciences*, vol. 83 (3): March, 1994, 296-299.

Gary Gagliardi, "Shark cartilage for achy joints." *Muscle and Fitness*, 56 (10), Oct. 1995, 52-57.

Kulkani, R.R., et al., "Treatment of osteoarthritis with a herbomineral formulation: A double-blind, placebo-controlled, cross-over study." *Journal of Ethnopharmacology*, (33), 1991, 91-95.

Lane, Dr. I. William and Linda Comac, *Sharks Don't Get Cancer*, (Avery Publishing, Garden City, New York: 1993), 117-20.

Merck Manual, 16th Edition, (Merck Research Laboratories, Rahway, New Jersey: 1992), 1338-1342.

Newman, M.N. and R.S.M. Ling, "Acetabular bone destruction related to nonsteroidal anti-inflammatory drugs." *Lancet*. II: 1985, 11. See also P.M. Brooks, et al., "NSAID and osteoarthritis, help or hindrance." *Journal of Rheumatology*. (9), 1982, 3-5.

Reichelt, A., et al., "Efficacy and safety of intramuscular glucosamine sulfate in osteoarthritis of the knee: A randomized, placebo-controlled, double-blind study." *Arneim-Forsch*. 44 (1), Jan. 1994, 75-80.

Rovetta, G., "Galactosaminoglycuronoglycan Sulfate (Matrix)in Therapy of Tibiofibular Osteoarthritis of the Knee," *Drugs in Experimental and Clinical Research*, 18 (1), 1991, 81-85.

Machtey and L. Ouaknine, "Tocopherol in osteoarthritis: A controlled pilot study," *Journal of the American Geriatrics Society*, (26), 1978, 328-30.

Schwartz, E.R., "The modulation of osteoarthritic development by vitamin C and E." *International Journal of Nutritional Research*, supplement, (26), 1984, 141-46.

Setnikar, I, et al., "Anti-arthritic effects of glucosamine sulfate studied in animal models." *Arneim-Forsch*. (41), 1991, 542-45.

Singh, G.B., et al., "Pharmacology of an extract of salai guggal ex-Boswellia serrata, a new nonsteroidal anti-inflammatory agent." *Agents Action*, (18), 1986, 407-12. See also Theodosakis, Jason, *The Arthritis Cure*, (St. Martin's Press, New York: 1997).

Travers, R.L., et al., "Boron and arthritis: The results of a double-blind pilot study." *Journal of Nutritional Medicine* (1), 1990. 127-32.

U.S. Patent #555569676, Inventor, Harry Weldon Diehl, Issue Date: October 29, 1996.

U.S. Patent #4,113,881, Inventor, Harry Weldon Diehl, Issue Date: September 12, 1978.

U.S. Patent #4,049,824, Inventor, Harry Weldon Diehl, Issue Date: September 20, 1977